About th

Rosita Evans qualified as a Fitness Instructor in 1986. She takes classes in London and is a personal trainer. Rosita also works with a local physiotherapy and sports injury practice, teaching yoga to patients as part of their recovery program.

Her love of dance and music is inherited from her father, a former ballroom and Latin American dance teacher. Her unusual Christian name comes from one of his favourite dances, a tango called 'Rosita'.

Rosita is interested in all aspects of health and fitness, especially complementary therapies. She is an avid reader and enjoys going to the cinema and theatre.

Born in London, Rosita now lives in Harrow, Middlesex.

Rosie's Armchair Exercises

A complete body workout, from the comfort of your own armchair

Rosita Evans

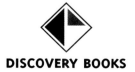

DISCOVERY BOOKS

First published in 2001 by Discovery Books
29 Hacketts Lane, Pyrford, Woking
Surrey GU22 8PP
Tel: 01932 400800
www.discoverybooks.co.uk
This edition published in 2012

A CIP catalogue record for this book is available
from the British Library.
ISBN 978-0-951851-17-3

Additional material and research by Catherine Beattie
Designed and typeset by David Simpson
Cover design by Sally Ann Thwaites

Printed and bound in Latvia by Dardedze Holography
www.dardedze.lv

Contents

Dedication

In memory of my oldest, dearest friend, Janet Taylor,
who lost her brave fight for life on
25 October 1999

Rest in peace, Jan.

Foreword

Many people consult their doctor with physical symptoms and problems that arise from a sedentary lifestyle, poor posture or simply a lack of exercise. These preventable symptoms include aches and pains, severe muscle stiffness and spasm, and lethargy.

Rosie's Armchair Exercises is a self-help manual aimed at helping many people attain a good level of physical fitness and mobility. The easy to follow text is well illustrated by clear pictures showing how to do the exercises correctly. All the exercises are presented in a logical, systematic way.

This book will clearly be useful for people who spend a lot of time sitting and provides a useful, easy method for improving and maintaining strength and mobility.

Rosita Evans has been extremely courageous and determined to maintain her own physical fitness. Through this book she offers others the opportunity to benefit from her experience.

Dr Mark L Levy, FRCGP
General Practitioner, Kenton, Middlesex, UK.

Introduction

Hello! My name is Rosie - Welcome to my 'Armchair Exercises' workout.

A few years ago I became ill with a chronic immune disorder. I had to drastically reduce the amount of exercise I was doing as I was finding it so tiring. It was at this point that I started devising my 'Armchair Exercises', purely for my own use. Over a period of time I experimented, added to my routine and soon felt the benefits. With relatively little physical effort, I was able to keep my body toned.

I now go through my Armchair Exercises at least twice a week. I was so delighted with the results that I began to think that many other people might also benefit from this form of exercise, and that is why I decided to write this book.

The program is designed for anyone who finds conventional exercising difficult - for example senior citizens, arthritis and rheumatism sufferers, and any-one with mobility problems or recuperating from ill-ness, injury or an operation.

The workout gently stretches the muscles of the body and helps keep the joints mobile. *All the exercises are carried out totally from the comfort of your armchair!* If done regularly over a period of time, you will become more flexible, and your muscles will be strengthened and toned. At no stage should the routine cause pain. If it does, then you must stop immediately. It is also important to stop whenever you wish to take a rest. Always listen to what your body is telling you and stop when you have had enough. After all, there is always tomorrow!

While these exercises are designed with safety of paramount importance throughout, it is always advisable to consult your doctor before embarking on any new exercise routine, and this one is no different.

To do these exercises you should be warm and comfortably seated in a chair with arms. Legs should be uncrossed and feet flat on the floor. If you have any problems with your lower back, put a small cushion between your lower back and the chair for added comfort.

Wear unrestricted, comfortable and loose clothing – a tracksuit, leggings or shorts are ideal. You will also need a rolled-up towel or small cushion to use during the leg section.

After a few weeks of doing the workout twice a week, you should be stronger and able to increase the repetitions in all sections.

I would advise you to read through the exercises at least once before attempting to do them.

Okay, let's start Rosie's Armchair Exercises...

Please note, exercises marked ✈ are also suitable for use by airline passengers and can be practised easily and discreetly from an aircraft seat. They help prevent the onset of deep vein thrombosis by maintaining healthy circulation in the legs and feet.
(See page 49 for more inflight exercises and tips on staying healthy when flying.)

Sitting up as straight as you can, take a deep cleansing breath in through your nostrils, and slowly let it out through your mouth. Repeat twice more.

We are going to start at the feet and work our way up through the body.

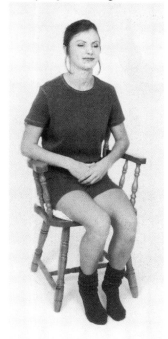

FEET and ANKLES

Stretches the Achilles tendon, helps eliminate swollen ankles and mobilises the ankle joint.

✈ Exercise 1

Pressing down onto the balls of both feet with heels lifted off the floor:

● Gently push the heels back down to the floor and then lift the heels up

● Repeat 4 times

✈ **Exercise 2**

Starting with the right foot:

● Lift the foot a few inches off the floor and point the toes down as far as possible

● *Hold for a count of 5*

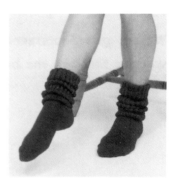

● Flex the foot (turn the toes upwards and push the heel down to the floor)

● *Hold for a count of 5*

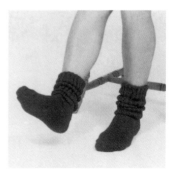

● Combine both movements and do 8 of each (4 points and 4 flexes) as quickly as possible

● Repeat with the left foot

✈ **Exercise 3**

Using the right foot and keeping the rest of the leg still:

● Lift the foot a couple of inches off the floor

● Gently rotate the ankle joint by drawing a circle with the toes

● Do 4 circles to the right

● Do 4 circles to the left

● Repeat with the left foot

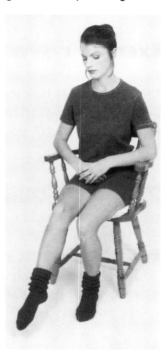

You may feel your thigh muscles working while doing these exercises – this is quite normal, because you are using them to hold your foot off the floor.

LEGS

(Stretches, lengthens and tones the muscles of the thighs and calves. Builds up the strength of the legs).

Exercise 1 - for the thigh muscles

This first exercise is in three parts, and is designed to warm up and stretch the thigh muscles.

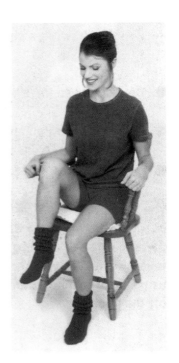

✈ **First part:**

Starting with the right leg:

● Lift the leg with the knee bent, as high as you can, taking care not to bend the body forward

● *Hold for a count of 8*

● Slowly bring the leg down again

● Repeat twice more (making three times in total), lifting the knee a little higher each time.

● Repeat with the left leg.

Second part:
With the right leg:

● Repeat the movement, and when the leg is lifted

● Straighten the leg as much as is comfortable

● Bend the knee and bring the foot gently down

● Repeat twice more (making three times in total)

● Repeat with left leg

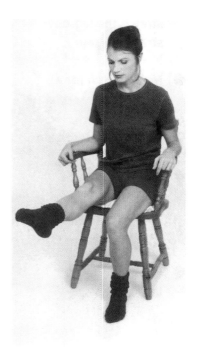

Third part:

With the right leg:

- Stretch the leg out in front

- Bend the knee very slightly and then stretch the leg out straight again

- *Hold stretch for a couple of seconds*

- Bend the knee again

- Repeat until you have done 10 'bend-stretches' in total

- Repeat with the left leg

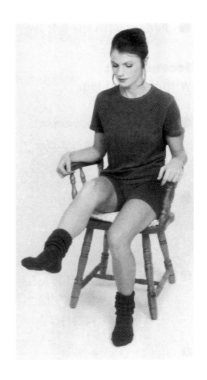

These movements should be done quite quickly. Make sure you keep the bend **very small**, and stretch the leg to your own maximum each time (holding the stretch for a couple of seconds). You should feel the front of the thigh muscle working.

Exercise 2 - for the calf muscles

Starting with the right leg:

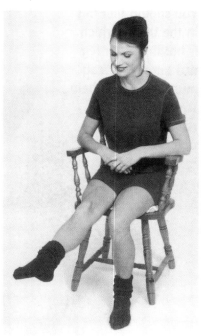

- Stretch the leg out in front (don't worry if you can only lift it a little way)

- Keeping the leg in this position, gently point the toes, then flex the foot so that the toes are facing up

- Do 8 sets of point/flexes and then lower the leg back down

- Repeat with the left leg

You should feel this in the thigh (which is holding your leg up) and in the calf muscle which is being stretched and relaxed by the point/flexing movement.

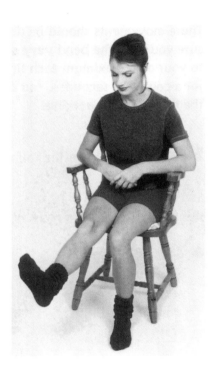

Exercise 3 - for the inside/outside thigh muscles:

Using the right leg:

- Lift the leg (as high as is comfortable) and stretch it out far as possible without locking the knee

- Slowly swing the leg out to the right as far as you can

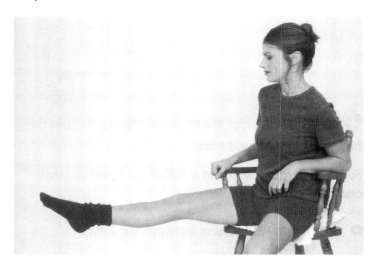

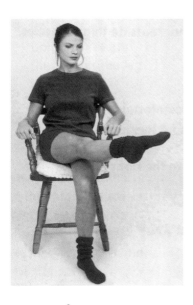

- Swing the leg back in and across your left leg as far as it goes

- Do this 4 times in all, and then rest (If you find this relatively easy, do another set of 4)

- Repeat with the left leg

Exercise 4 - for the inside thigh muscles, working both legs at the same time.

For this exercise you need a rolled-up towel or small cushion:

- Grip the towel/cushion between the knees

- Squeeze the knees together, gripping the towel/cushion tightly

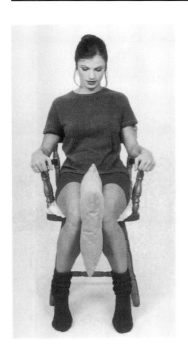 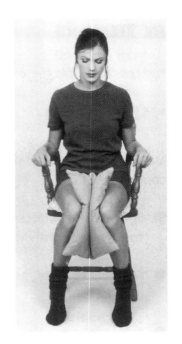

● Squeeze for a count of 3

● Relax slightly for just a second

● Squeeze again for a count of 3

● Repeat 8 times

BOTTOM

Tightens and lifts the buttock muscles.

✈ **Exercise 1**

Make sure you are still sitting comfortably:

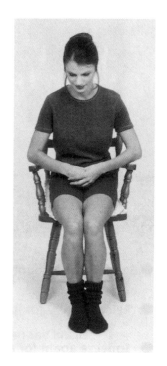

● Squeeze the buttocks together as tightly possible

● *Hold the squeeze for a slow count of 3*

● Release the muscles and immediately squeeze again for a count of 3

Aim to do this at times to start with, more if you can manage it – the more you do, the tighter your bottom will become! If you are squeezing hard, you should feel yourself 'lift' slightly.

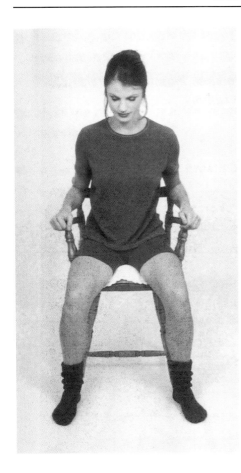

Exercise 2

Once you have mastered Exercise 1, the same exercise can be done sitting with the legs as wide apart as possible.

You will find it is much more difficult to squeeze the buttocks together in this position, which makes the muscles work harder!

ABDOMEN

Strengthens the abdominal muscles and helps to flatten and tone the tummy.

Exercise 1

You should still be sitting comfortably:

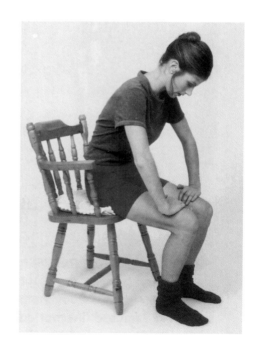

- Lean forward slightly, placing the hands on the thighs

- Take a deep breath in through the nose

● Breathing out through the mouth, pull the tummy muscles in tightly (imagine you are trying to get your navel to touch your spine)

● *Hold the position for a few seconds, **breathing normally***

● Relax and take another breath in through the nostrils

● Breath out through the mouth and repeat pulling in the tummy muscles

Do this exercise 5 times to start with, gradually increasing the repetitions as you build up strength. It is a good way of toning and flattening the abdominal muscles, so persevere!

The following routine takes the exercise a stage further and uses the muscles in the waist, which are part of the abdominal muscles (the obliques).

Exercise 2

Sitting up straight in the chair:

- Turn the body to the right

- Place both hands on the right arm of the chair

- Lean forward, keeping the body turned to the right

- Repeat exercise 1 in this position

- Repeat turning to the left

Once you have mastered this stomach exercise, you may like to try another one.

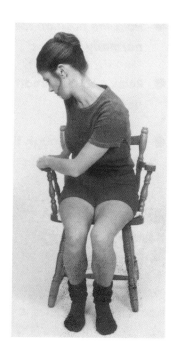

Exercise 3

Slide your bottom towards the edge of your chair.
Push the lower back into the seat and keep it 'glued'
there throughout the exercise:

● Grip the arms of the chair firmly

● Breathe out and bring the knees into the chest

● Breathe in and
take the feet back
down to the floor

Try to do this exercise
5 times to start with,
bringing the knees
as close as possible
to the chest each
time. The exercise
should be done at
your own speed,
but do remember
the breathing
instructions.

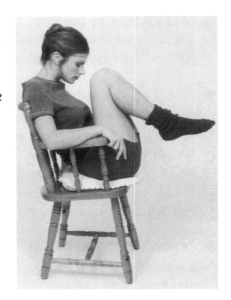

SPINE STRETCH

Keeps the spine mobile and eases back ache.

Sitting up as straight as possible, arms to your sides, hands on the chair:

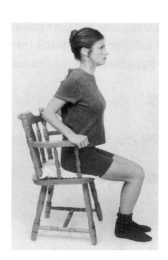

- Take a deep breath and arch the back by pushing the bottom out and holding the shoulders back

- Slowly breathe out as you reverse the movement by rounding the spine towards the back of the chair and bringing the shoulders down and forward

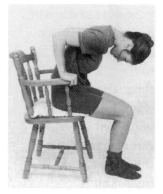

- Repeat both movements at a comfortable pace until you have done 5 sets

WAIST STRETCH

Stretches and tones the waist and midriff area.

Keeping the body upright with the bottom and thighs on the chair:

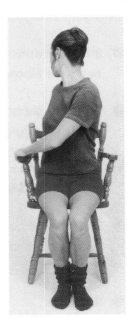

● Turn the upper body to the right, placing both hands firmly on the right arm of the chair

● *Hold this position, breathing gently, for a few seconds*

● Edge round a little further (keep firmly anchored to the chair and do not lean forwards)

● *Hold the position for 30 seconds* before returning to the front

● Repeat to the left side.

You should feel a pull in your waist area as it is being stretched.

PECTORAL (chest wall) MUSCLE

Strengthens the chest wall muscle and improves the appearance of the bust. In men it firms up flabby tissue and develops 'firm pecs'.

Sitting up straight:

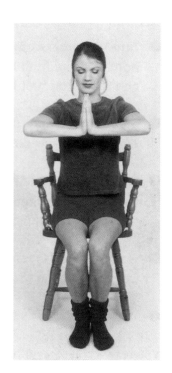

- Bring the arms up and bend the elbows

- Press the palms of the hands together in the 'praying' position (keep the elbows high and out to the sides)

- Squeeze the heels of the hands together as firmly as possible

- Release

- Repeat

You should feel the pectoral muscle (under the arms and to the sides of the chest) working.
Aim to do 30 sets to start with at a pace of one squeeze per second. When you can do this comfortably, do an additional set of 15 as follows:

● *Hold the squeeze for a slow count of 3*

● Release and repeat.

UPPER ARMS

Tightens and strengthens the upper arms.

Exercise 1

Sitting up straight:

● Stretch the arms
straight out in front
with the palms
facing down

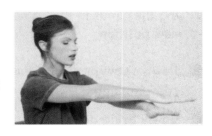

● Criss-cross the hands over and under each other,
keeping the arms straight

- Criss-cross the hands as quickly as possible, keeping the movement small and tight (only use the hands – not the whole arms)

- Slowly begin raising the arms up, still criss-crossing

- Slowly bring down, still criss-crossing

- Repeat 3 times

- Without pausing and keeping the arms straight, turn the palms upwards

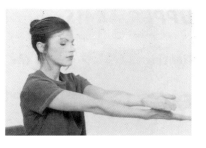

- Continue criss-crossing the hands in the new position

- Slowly raise the arms as high as possible, still criss-crossing

- Slowly bring down, still criss-crossing

- Repeat 3 times

Exercise 2

● Take the arms out to the sides

● Straighten arms and clench both fists

● Using both arms, start making small circling motions using the whole arm (Do this quite quickly and keep the circles small)

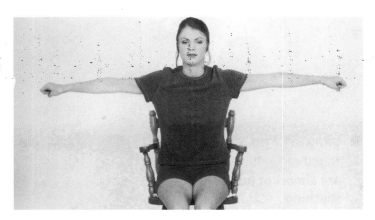

● Circle one way for a count of 10

● Circle the other way for a count of 10

● Repeat twice more (making three sets in total)

SHOULDERS

Keeps the shoulder joints rotating freely.

Exercise 1

● Place the hands lightly on the shoulders

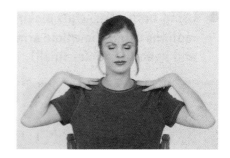

● Bring the elbows together so they are almost or just touching

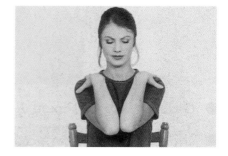

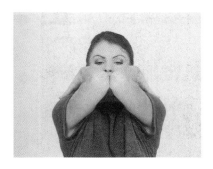

● Keeping the elbows together, raise them up in front as high as possible

● Open out to the sides with a big circular movement

● Bring the elbows back down to the starting position

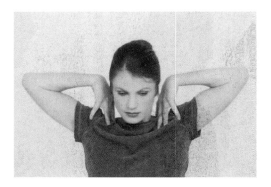

● Repeat slowly twice more

This exercise rotates the shoulder joints through their maximum range. If you find it difficult, maybe because you cannot reach your shoulders with your hands, try the following exercise instead. This also fully rotates the shoulders.

Exercise 2

● Rest the hands lightly on the top of the thighs

● Keeping the body still, make gentle backward
circling motions with the shoulders

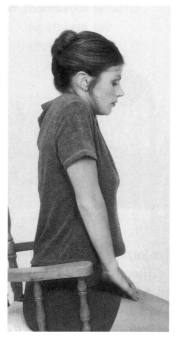
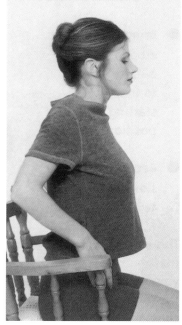

- Gradually make the circles as large as is comfortable

- Slowly decrease the size of the circles

The whole exercise should take about a minute.
The circles should be in a backwards direction and not forwards, as this may encourage round shoulders

NECK

Loosens the neck muscles, eliminating stress and stiffness from the neck area.

Exercise 1

Sitting up straight, with the face looking directly forwards and not tilted down:

- Breathing normally, slowly turn the head to the **left**

- *Hold for a count of 5* (keeping the chin level and shoulders back)

- Slowly bring the head back to the original position

- Turn the head to the **right**

- *Hold for a count of 5*

- Repeat twice

- Do a further 3 sets without the 5 count pause, so there is continuous movement.

Exercise 2

Sitting up straight:

- Gently let the chin fall down to the chest as low as is comfortable

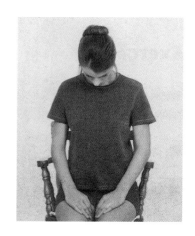

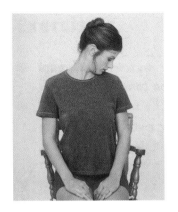 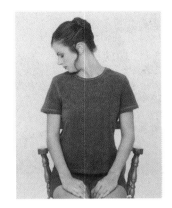

- Slowly rotate the head to the **left** shoulder and **no further**

- Let the chin drop down again

- Slowly rotate the head to the **right** shoulder

- Repeat 4 more times, making 5 in all

- This exercise should always be done slowly. **Never** attempt to fully rotate your head in this position, as such a movement is likely to trap nerves and harm the delicate neck vertebrae.

FACE

Facial exercises gently work the muscles just under the skin surface, to keep the face toned.

Exercise 1

Sitting comfortably:

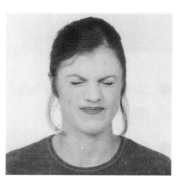

● Close the eyes

● Screw the face up as much as possible

● Open the eyes and mouth wide

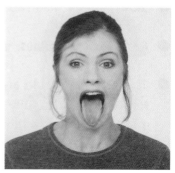

● Breathe out and stick out the tongue to its furthest extent

● *Hold for a count of 5*

● Repeat

Exercise 2

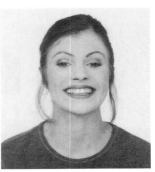

● Relax the face

● Looking straight ahead, raise the eyebrows as high as possible

● *Hold for a count of 5*

● Repeat twice more

Exercise 3

● Relax the face

● Purse the lips, pushing them forward as much as possible

● Pull the lips back into a wide open grin and **hold for a count of 5**

● Repeat twice

Exercise 4

● Relax the face

● Purse the lips

● Keeping the lips pursed, move lips to the right
(as if trying to touch the ear).

● Move lips to the left

● Repeat to each side five times.

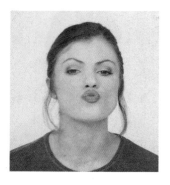 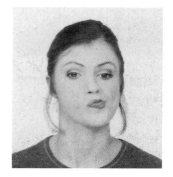

Exercise 5

● Relax the face

● Close the mouth

● Push out the lower jaw as far as it will go.

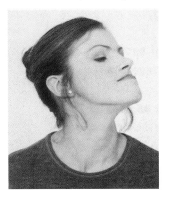

● *Hold for a count of 5.*

● Repeat twice more.

If you find this relatively easy, try tilting the head back **slightly** for more effect.

✈ *And to finish...*

Sitting up straight,
take a deep breath in
through the nostrils
and stretch the arms up
towards the ceiling,
linking the hands
together.

Stretch up as much as
feels comfortable,
then gently let the arms
come down as you
breathe out through
your mouth.
Repeat twice more.

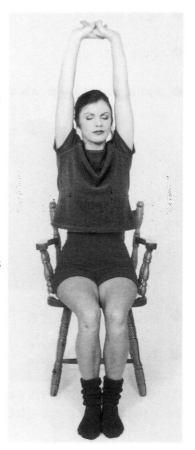

Well done!

You have now completed Rosie's Armchair Exercises!
From the comfort of your own armchair, you have
exercised the whole of your body. Although you have
been sitting down throughout, do not think you have
not worked hard. You have, and as a result may even
feel a little stiff tomorrow.

If you do this routine two or three times a week, you
will soon notice a gradual improvement in your muscle
strength and tone.

As you get used to the exercises, try to increase the
number of repetitions so that you are working harder.
This will make the good results even more pronounced.

Good luck, and stay fit!

✈ ARMCH**AIR** EXERCISES ✈

During the preparation of this book, the health risks of air travel have been in the news. Passengers are in danger of developing deep vein thrombosis (DVT) — a blood clot — as a result of dehydration and sitting in cramped conditions for long periods of time. This may have fatal consequences if the clot is carried along in the bloodstream and blocks the vital blood supply to the heart, lungs or brain. Yet, by taking a few simple precautions, the condition can usually be prevented.

Even if you have flown trouble-free for years, it does not mean you are 'immune' to the problem of DVT, as the risk occurs every time you fly. Long haul flights are the most hazardous, although the condition has been known to occur on flights as short as two hours. That said, developing a blood clot during or after a flight is still a relatively rare event, so try not to worry. Just be aware of the danger and minimise your risk by drinking extra water and fluids, walking up and down the aisles at regular intervals and doing the following inflight exercises. Prevention is always better than cure!

Several exercises in this book are ideal for use by air travellers — just read 'aircraft seat' for 'armchair'. All are designed to boost circulation in the lower limbs, where inflight blood clots are most likely to develop. These exercises help to minimise pooling of blood in the veins and tissues of the legs, ankles and feet and are easily carried out at any time when sitting in your seat. Do not be fooled by their simplicity — practised regularly during a flight they will reduce your risk of developing a blood clot.

A combination of armch**AIR** exercises, stretching your legs in the aisles and drinking extra water and fluids will ensure your flight is as risk-free as possible. These safeguards should be routine every time you fly.

Page 13 Feet/Ankles

All exercises in this section are particularly beneficial. You should be able to do them without difficulty even in a confined space. A further advantage is that they help prevent swollen ankles, another (more common and less serious) side-effect of flying.

Page 16 Legs (thighs/calf muscles)

You can easily do the first part of this exercise, but will not have enough space for the second and third parts.

Instead, try 'quick marching' on the spot. Lift your knees as high as you can manage comfortably and try to keep marching for at least a minute. This is a good way of relieving compression on the veins at the back of the upper leg by the edge of the seat.

 ## Page 24 Bottom

The first exercise (squeezing and releasing the buttock muscles) is easily carried out in the confines of your aircraft seat. Like the other exercises, it tones the muscles (of the pelvic floor) and aids circulation.

 ## Page 46 ....And to finish

End your short routine with a lovely long stretch, arms in the air and fingers linked, as you reach up as high as you can. Don't forget to breathe in deeply as you do this, then exhale, as you slowly bring your arms down. Inhaling and exhaling fully and deeply is particularly beneficial in the rarefied atmosphere of the cabin. The extra intake of oxygen improves concentration and keeps you feeling alert.

Ideally, the whole of this simple routine — which takes only minutes — should be done hourly. Aim to drink a glass of water after completing each session.

Self-help guidelines to ensure a safe and enjoyable journey each time you fly

✔ If you are due to fly and think you may be particularly susceptible to developing a blood clot (perhaps you or other members of your family have had one previously, or you have recently had surgery or take medications that increase your risk, including HRT and the Pill), please see your doctor. You may need to be prescribed blood-thinning drugs and/or special support stockings to wear during the flight. These are much tighter than ordinary stockings and designed to support the leg veins and aid blood flow.

✔ Drink extra water and fluids on the days before you fly and have a good night's sleep prior to departure. Do not exhaust yourself doing last minute jobs before heading for the airport. You are more likely to fly trouble-free if you arrive rested and in good time for your flight.

✔ Wear loose and comfortable clothing in layers that you can take off and put on during the flight. Avoid anything restrictive or tight.

✔ Take aspirin — it is not just for headaches! As well as being an effective painkiller, aspirin has blood-thinning properties that stop formation of blood clots. Doctors have prescribed aspirin for years to prevent heart attacks and strokes in patients known to be at risk. A single tablet taken for just three days (the day before your flight, the day of your flight and one day after) could be of great benefit. Check with your doctor if you have any doubts about self-dosing, as aspirin is not suitable for everyone.

✘ The cabin atmosphere is drier than a desert and on long flights you will suffer cracked lips, dry skin, itchy eyes, and may feel lightheaded or queasy. Overcome these problems by packing moisturiser, vaseline (for lips and nostrils), eyedrops and a small Evian spray in your carry-on bag. Ginger capsules are an effective remedy for nausea. More seriously, dry cabin air may exacerbate inflight dehydration — a real threat to health because it makes the blood stickier and more likely to clot.

✔ Drinking plenty of fluids, particularly water and fruit juice is the best way to counteract dehydration. Always have a glass of water in front of you and drink one large glass (preferably more) every hour. Aircraft carry limited amounts of water, so bring your own bottled supply and take regular sips. Limit your intake of tea, coffee and caffeinated soft drinks because they have diuretic properties and ultimately make you even more dehydrated. Better to quench your thirst with frequent drinks of water and fruit juice.

✗ Although few airlines discourage inflight drinking, alcohol and flying are incompatible travelling companions — rather like drinking and driving. A little alcohol may be relaxing, but its dehydrating effects increase your risk of developing blood clots. Some people find that even a small amount of inflight alcohol makes them feel faint and unwell (alcohol affects blood pressure levels and impairs how the body utilises oxygen). Remember, one drink in the air is worth two on the ground. You become intoxicated quicker on a pressurised jet than drinking in an airport bar.

✔ Recent research suggests that a light snack and a non-alcoholic drink consumed **before you board,** lowers your risk of a heart attack or fainting during the flight. A *small* meal increases the circulating blood volume, helping maintain blood pressure and oxygen levels and easing your adjustment to the pressurised cabin environment.

✗ Low pressure cabin air contains less oxygen than air on the ground, so during a long flight the body's oxygen levels fall and most passengers experience a mild degree of hypoxia (oxygen deprivation). The signs include shallow breathing, fatigue, an inability to concentrate and feeling clammy and faint. If you start feeling ill or uncomfortably hot, tell a flight attendant you are unwell and need the flow of fresh (oxygenated) air into the cabin increased (the pilot may have reduced it to save fuel). You will soon recover when the air quality improves. (First class passengers at the front of the aircraft enjoy three times more air than economy passengers, so rarely encounter this problem.)

If you ever have difficulty breathing when flying, call a flight attendant immediately and ask for an oxygen bottle. You will be shown how to use it and feel better after a few breaths. All planes carry oxygen and such emergencies are not uncommon.

✗ Do not sit or sleep with your legs crossed as this restricts blood flow through the leg veins. Avoid any type of obstruction near or around the calves when sitting and do not sleep with any constriction on your lower legs. Ease compression on the veins at back of the upper legs by placing your feet on a bag or leg rest for short periods.

✔ Stand up and walk around the cabin as often as possible (even if you have to squeeze past sleeping passengers). Your increased fluid intake not only prevents you becoming dehydrated but ensures you take exercise too — with multiple trips to the lavatory!

✔ Finally, an effective exercise to do whenever you are out of your seat.

- *Stand up.*
- *Go right up onto your toes*
- *Lower your heels to a standing position*

Aim to do **twenty** of these heel lifts on an hourly basis, as quickly as you can manage. They really pep up circulation in the lower leg and are easily carried out while waiting in that inevitable queue!

Happy landings!

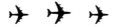

Healthy flying checklist

Before boarding
❑ Take aspirin ❑ Drink extra fluids ❑ Eat a small meal

On board
Tick the boxes in these charts to remind you to exercise
regularly and to drink extra water during your flight.

Hours into flight	Armch**AIR** exercises	Drink a glass of water	Stretch legs in aisle
One			
Two			
Three			
Four			
Five			
Six			
Seven			
Eight			
Nine			
Ten			
Eleven			
Twelve			
Thirteen			
Fourteen			

Healthy flying checklist

Hours into flight	Armch*AIR* exercises	Drink a glass of water	Stretch legs in aisle
One			
Two			
Three			
Four			
Five			
Six			
Seven			
Eight			
Nine			
Ten			
Eleven			
Twelve			
Thirteen			
Fourteen			

Healthy flying checklist

Hours into flight	Armch*AIR* exercises	Drink a glass of water	Stretch legs in aisle
One			
Two			
Three			
Four			
Five			
Six			
Seven			
Eight			
Nine			
Ten			
Eleven			
Twelve			
Thirteen			
Fourteen			

Meet the team

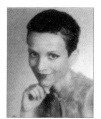

Rosita Evans
Author

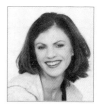

Sarah Beattie
Model

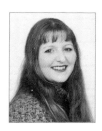

Nadine McKenney
Stylist

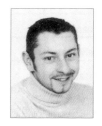

Stephen Aspinall
Photographer